A DAY IN THE LIFE OF A COMMUNITY SERVICE VEHICLE

A DAY IN THE LIFE OF AN AMBULANCE

by Mae Respicio

PEBBLE
a capstone imprint

Published by Pebble, an imprint of Capstone
1710 Roe Crest Drive, North Mankato, Minnesota 56003
capstonepub.com

Copyright © 2025 by Capstone. All rights reserved. No part of this publication may be reproduced in whole or in part, or stored in a retrieval system, or transmitted in any form or by any means, electronic, mechanical, photocopying, recording, or otherwise, without written permission of the publisher.

Library of Congress Cataloging-in-Publication Data is available on the Library of Congress website.
ISBN: 9780756587222 (hardcover)
ISBN: 9780756587178 (paperback)
ISBN: 9780756587185 (ebook PDF)

Summary: An ambulance speeds by on its way to an emergency. Crews depend on ambulances to help them care for people. What equipment is in an ambulance? How do ambulance crews make sure their vehicles are ready for the day? Find out how workers use ambulances from sunrise to sunset.

Editorial Credits
Editor: Carrie Sheely; Designer: Elyse White; Media Researcher: Jo Miller; Production Specialist: Tori Abraham

Image Credits
Getty Images: Fotografía de eLuVe, 11, Halfpoint Images, 12, kali9, 19, majorosl, 14, 15, Tammy Hanratty/Corbis/VCG, 5, 7, tillsonburg, 16; Shutterstock: Bojan Pesic, cover (front and back), blurAZ, 4, Matt Gush, 13, My Ocean Production, 9, Nuttapong, 20 (paper), Pitchayarat Chootai, 20 (pencils), Seth Gallmeyer, 6, Stefan Malloch, 18, Tyler Olson, 17, yanchi1984, 21

Any additional websites and resources referenced in this book are not maintained, authorized, or sponsored by Capstone. All product and company names are trademarks™ or registered® trademarks of their respective holders.

TABLE OF CONTENTS

Emergency Vehicles 4
A Sunrise Start 6
A Day of Helping 12
Sunset at the Hospital 18
    Ambulance Artwork 20
    Glossary 22
    Read More 23
    Internet Sites 23
    Index 24
    About the Author 24

Words in **bold** are in the glossary.

EMERGENCY VEHICLES

Wee-ooh! Wee-ooh! Look! An ambulance speeds down the road. Ambulances are **emergency** vehicles. They bring injured and sick people to hospitals. **Paramedics** and **emergency medical technicians** (EMTs) are workers who use ambulances.

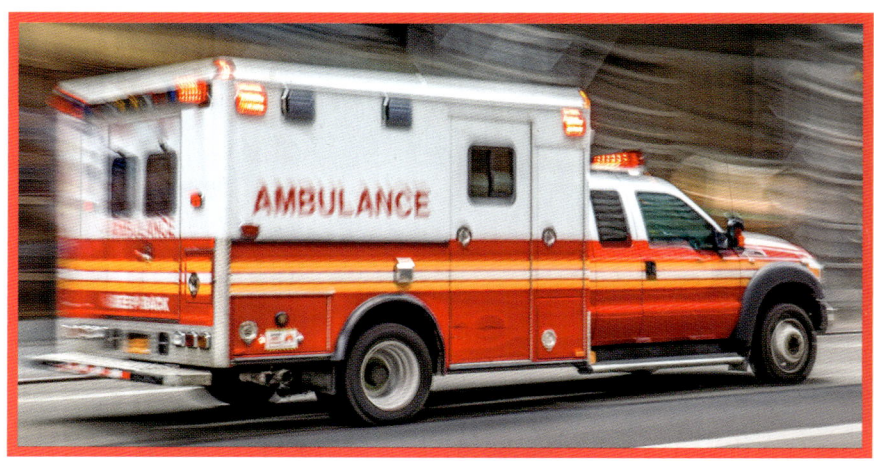

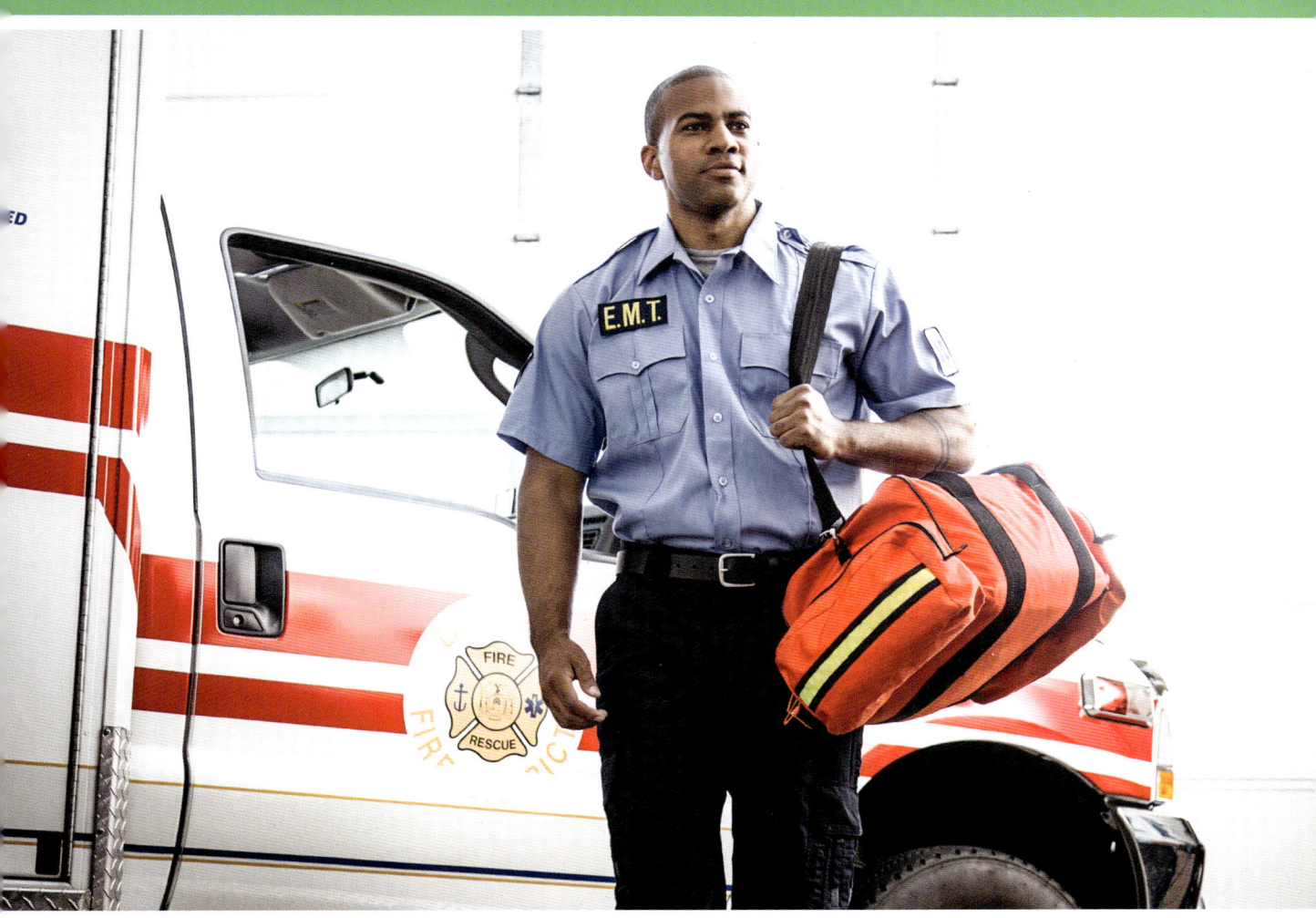

A SUNRISE START

It's sunrise. A crew gets to the ambulance station. It is at a **community** hospital. The ambulances are parked there.

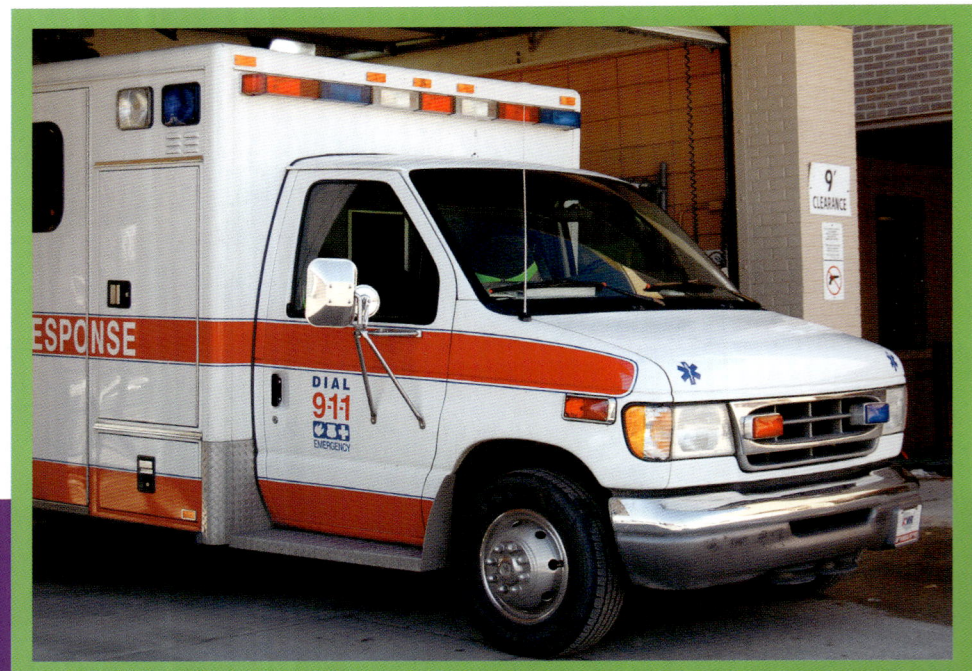

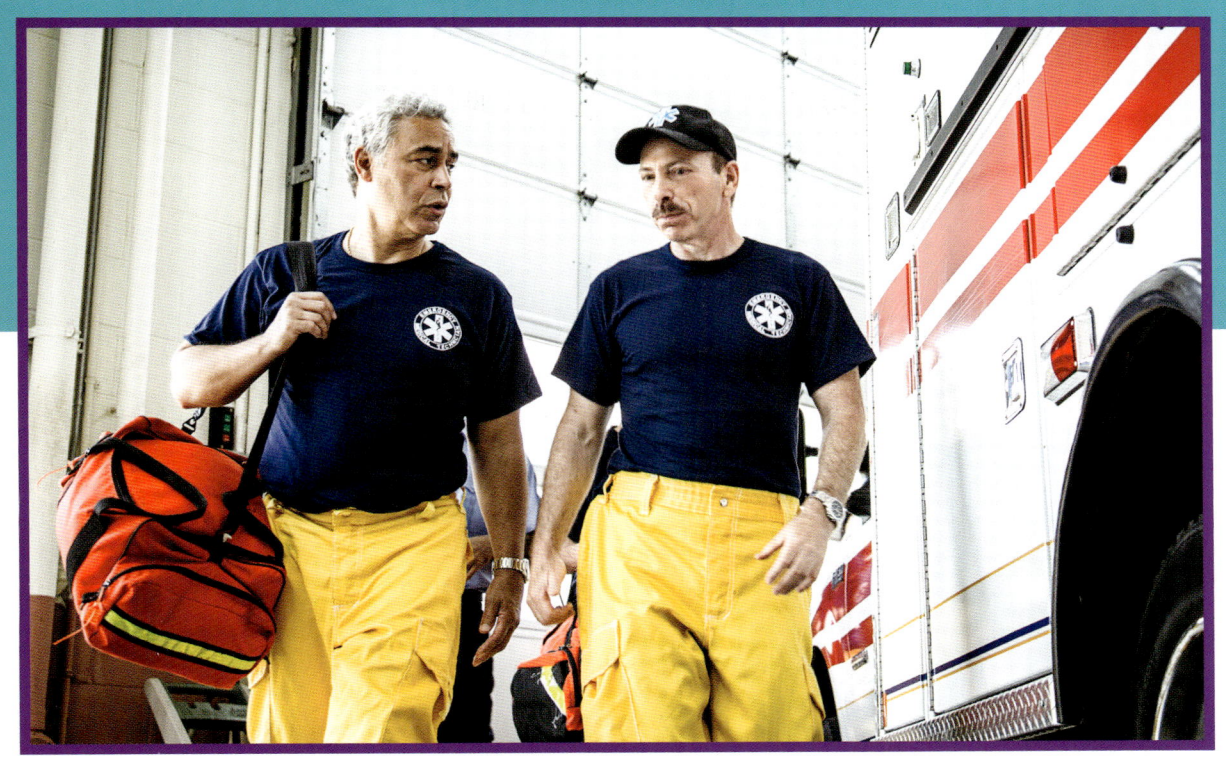

An ambulance usually has at least two workers. One person drives. The other person helps **patients** in the back of the vehicle.

The workers open the ambulance's back doors. What's inside? A lot of equipment! Some patients may be having a hard time breathing. **Ventilators** can give them air. There is a bed called a **stretcher**. Cabinets hold medicine and other supplies.

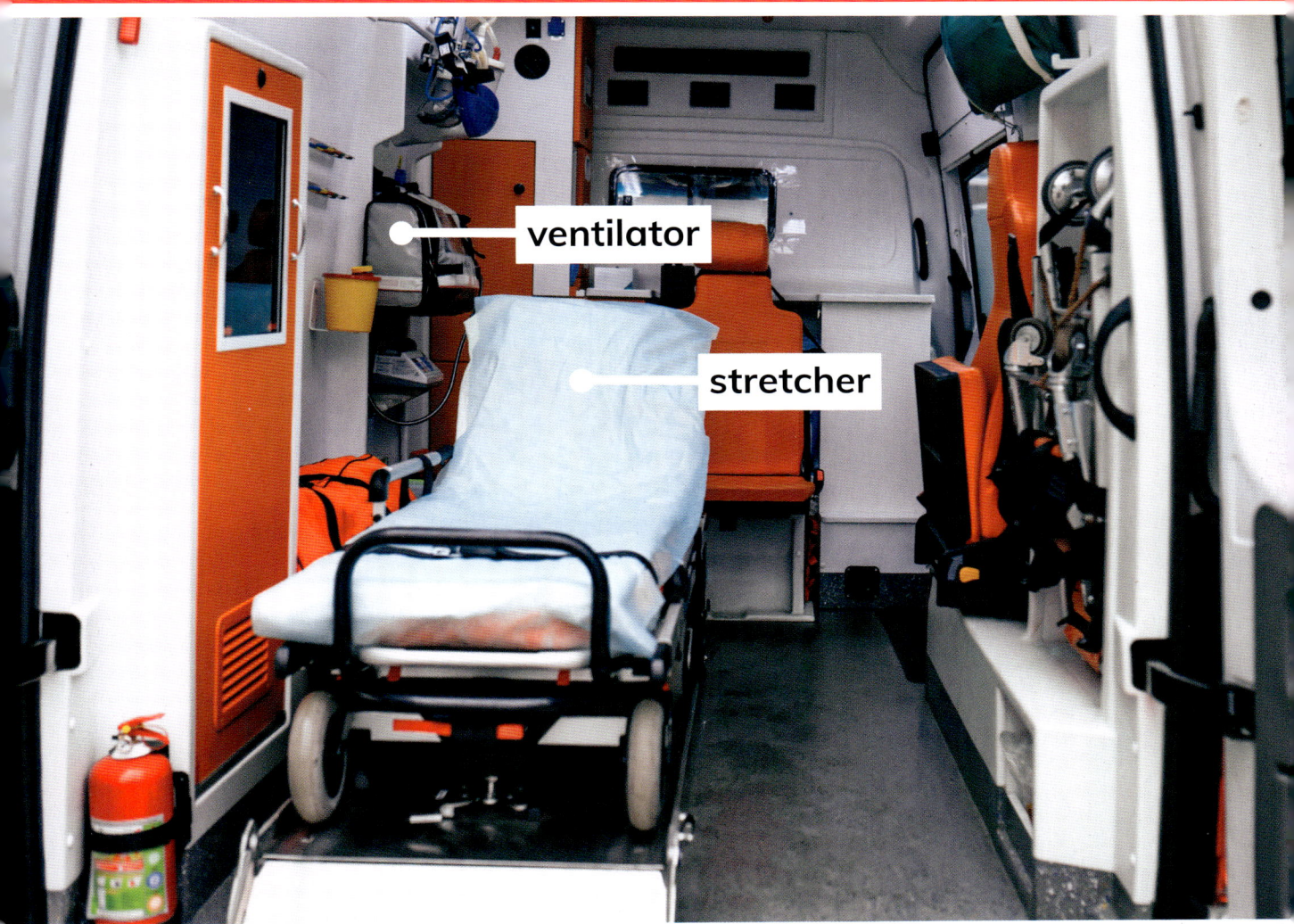

Crews make sure all the gear is organized. They check that nothing is missing. They make sure equipment batteries are charged.

Workers check the ambulance too. Do the lights work? Is there enough **fuel**? Are the tires in good shape? Yes! Now the ambulance is ready to go.

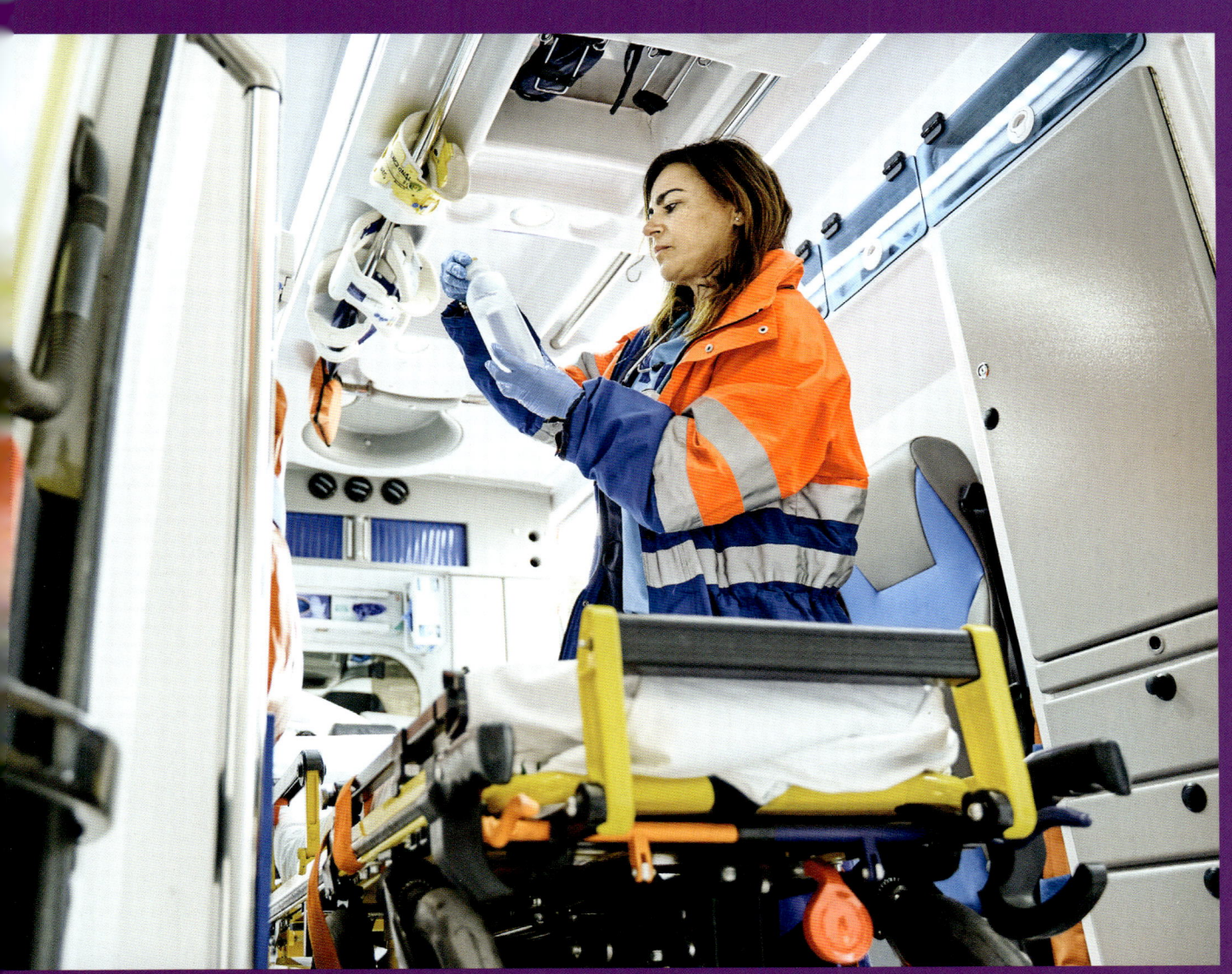

A DAY OF HELPING

Beep! The crew hears the **dispatcher** talk over the radio. Someone nearby needs help.

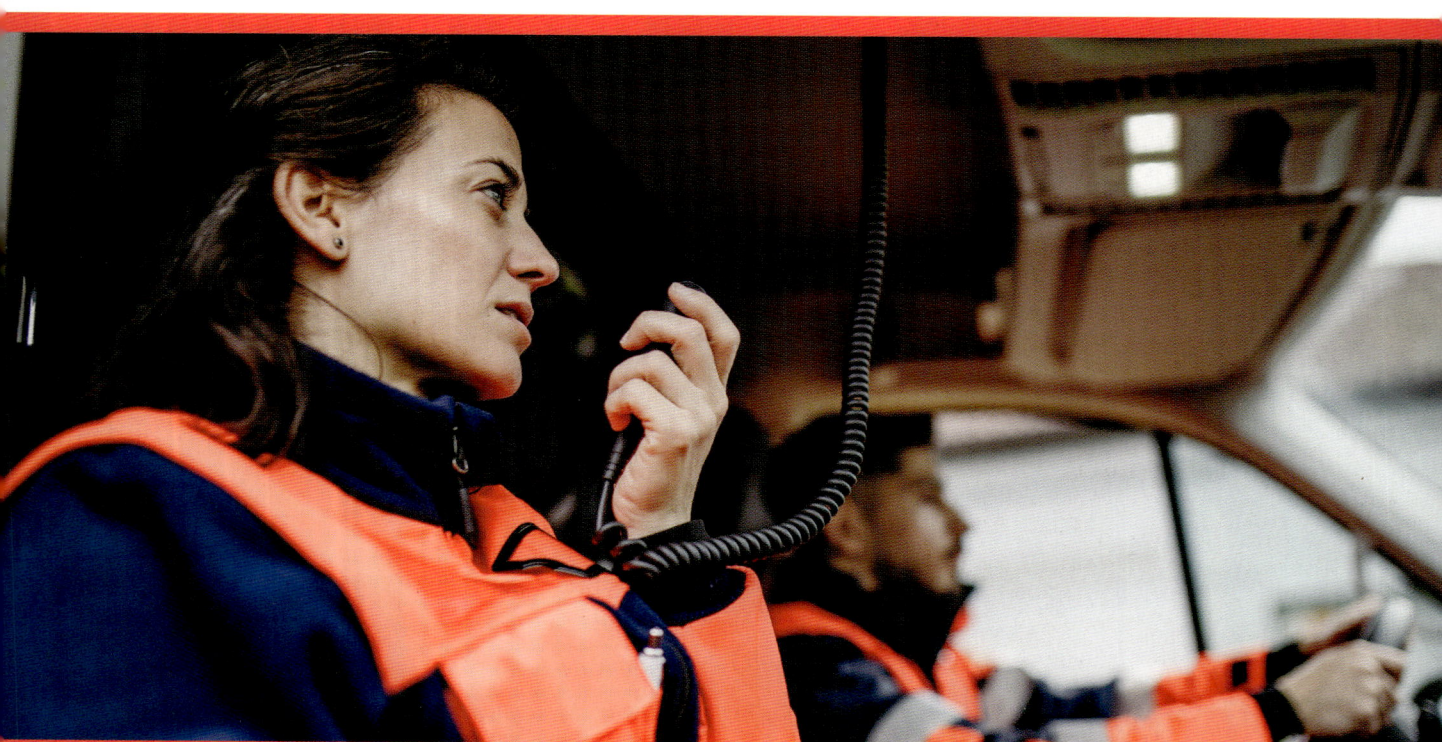

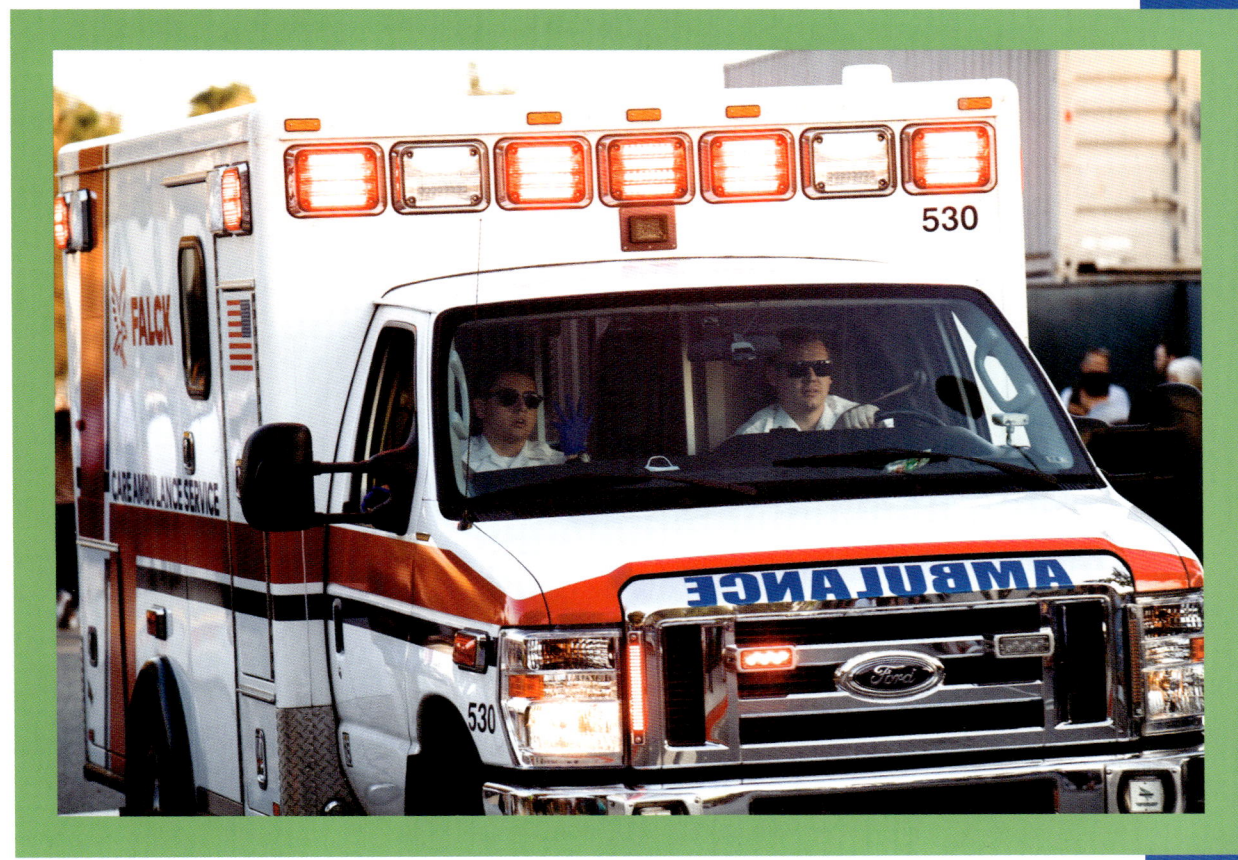

The ambulance springs into action. Its lights flash. The siren wails. The ambulance rushes through traffic. Cars pull over to move out of the way.

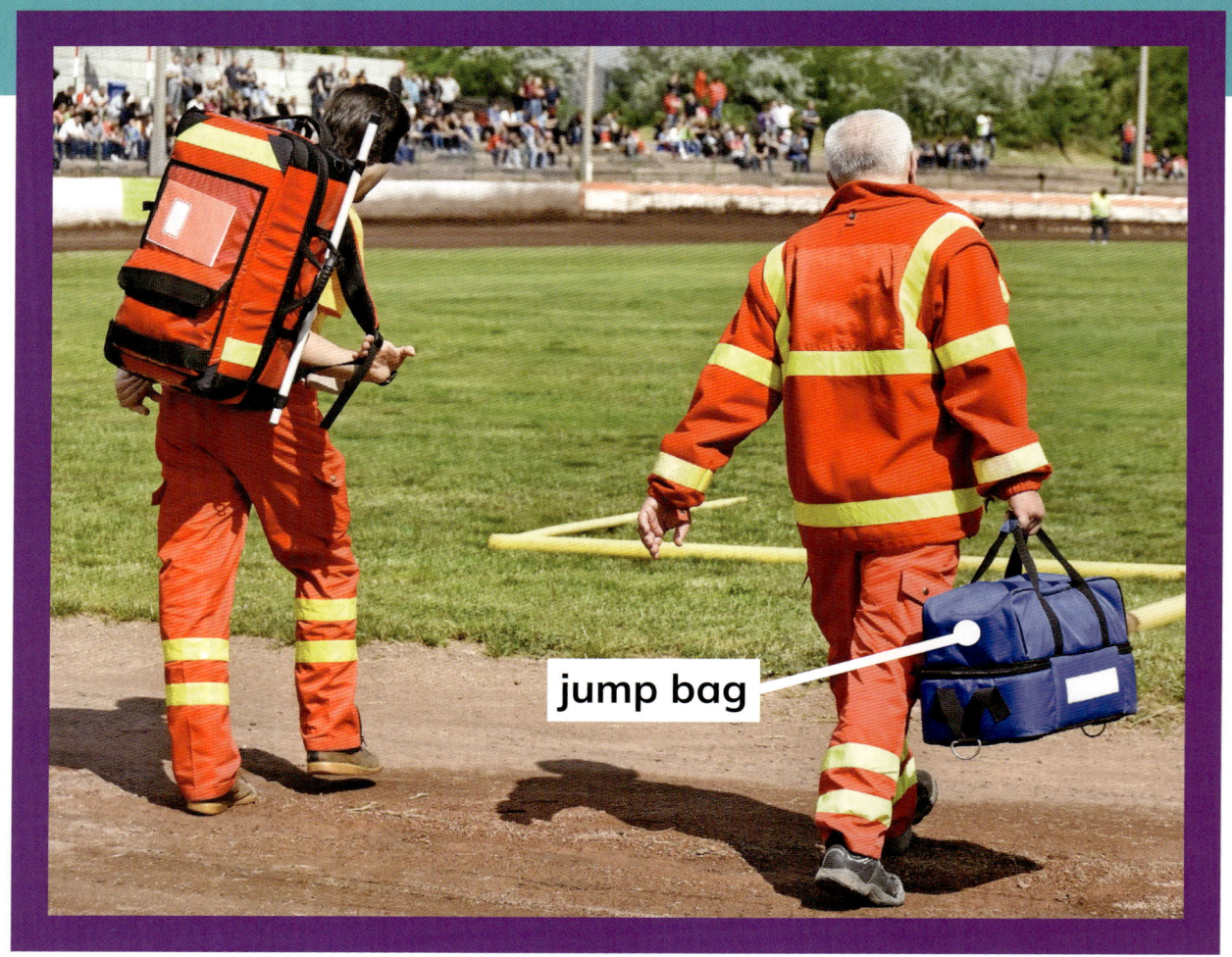

The crew arrives at a sports event. The ambulance pulls up as close as possible to the patient. The workers grab their jump bag.

A player has hurt their leg. The workers care for the patient. They ask questions about what happened. Then they decide if the person needs hospital care.

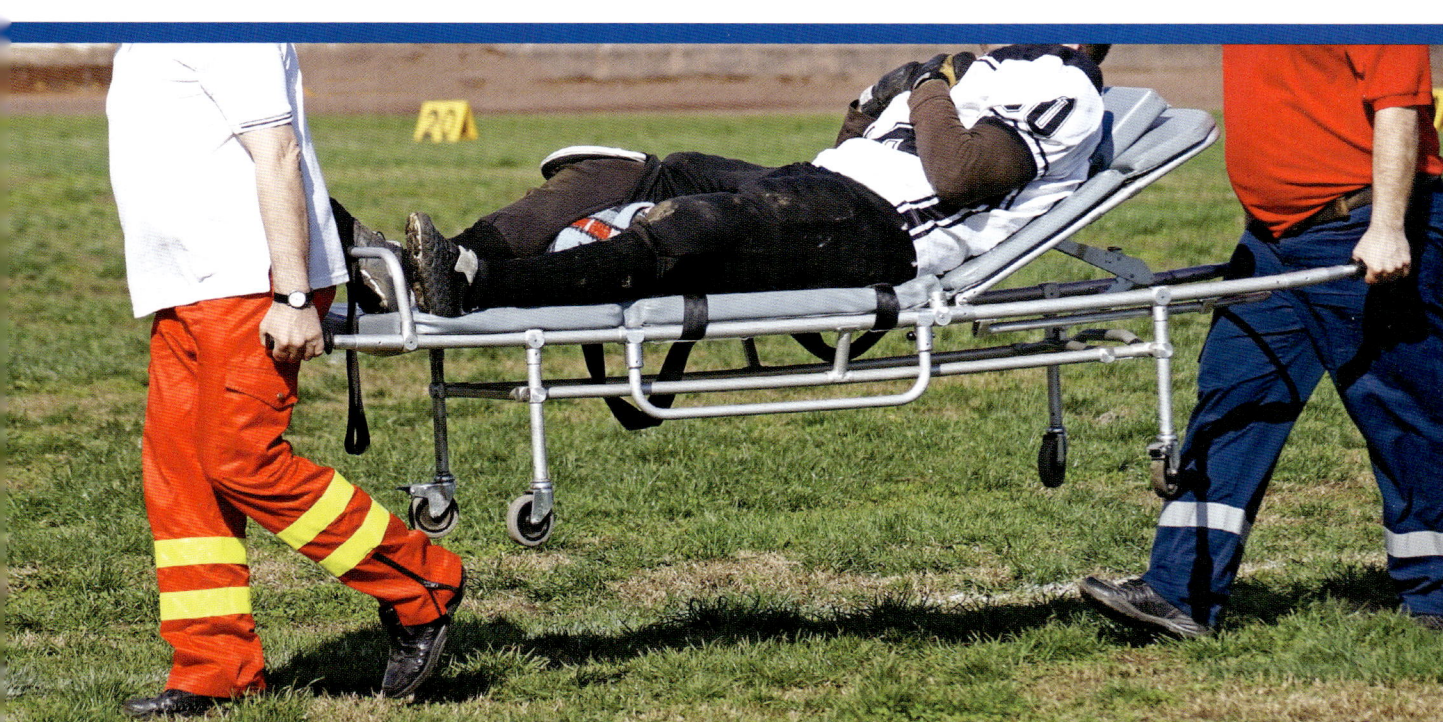

Soon, the ambulance crew gets another call. There was a car accident. *Zoom!* The ambulance speeds to the scene.

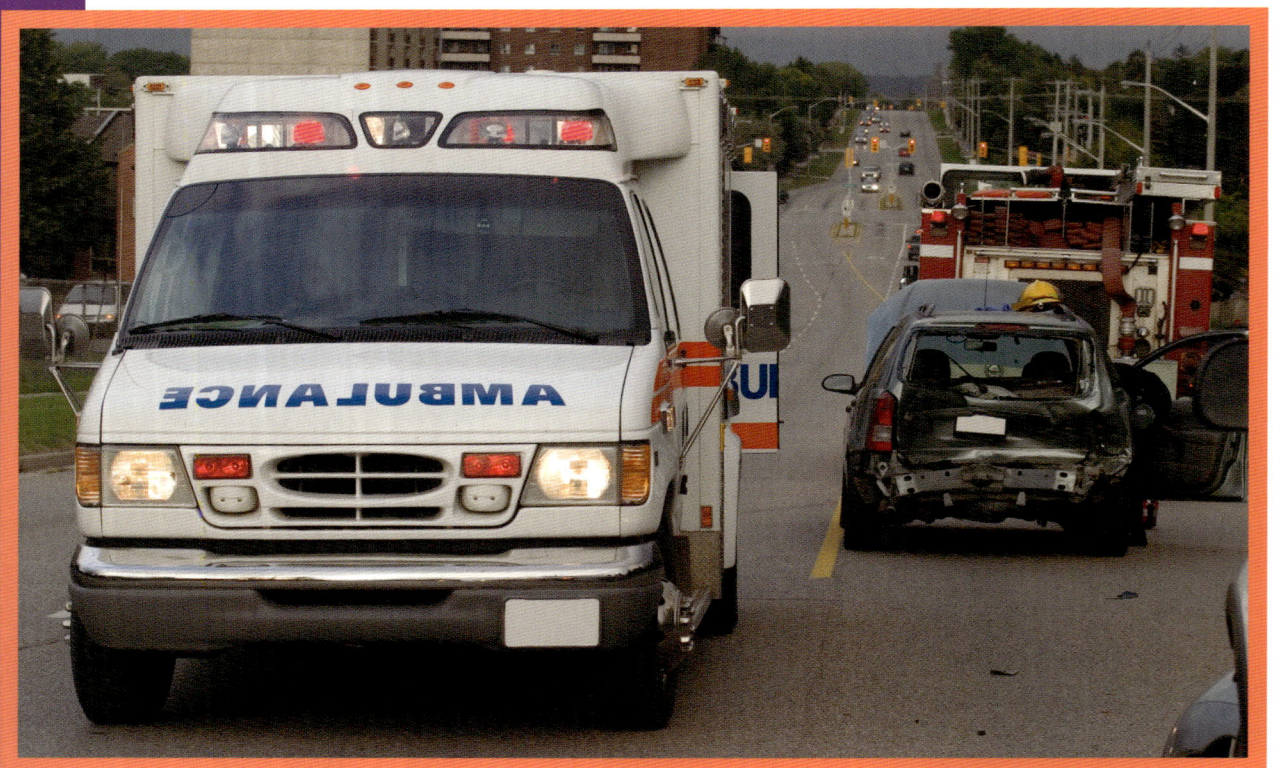

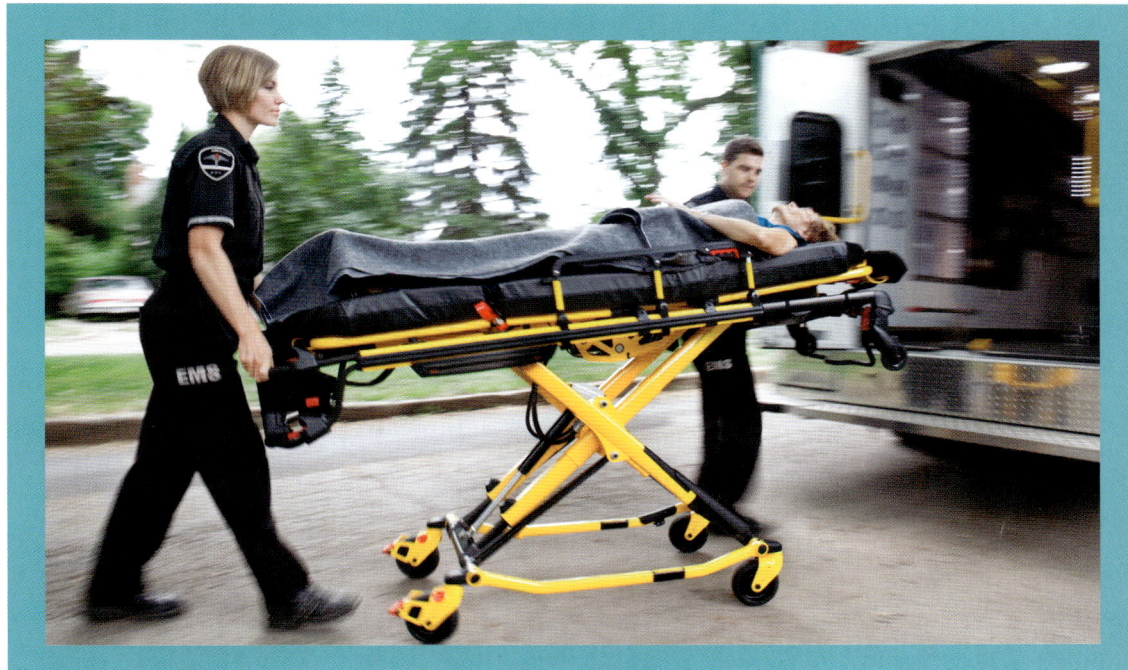

The crew checks on people needing help.
One person might have a broken bone.
Do they need to go to the hospital? Yes.
The crew helps the patient onto a stretcher.
It is lifted into the ambulance.

SUNSET AT THE HOSPITAL

The ambulance zips to the hospital. Carefully, the workers lift out the stretcher. They bring the patient inside. Now the hospital crew takes over.

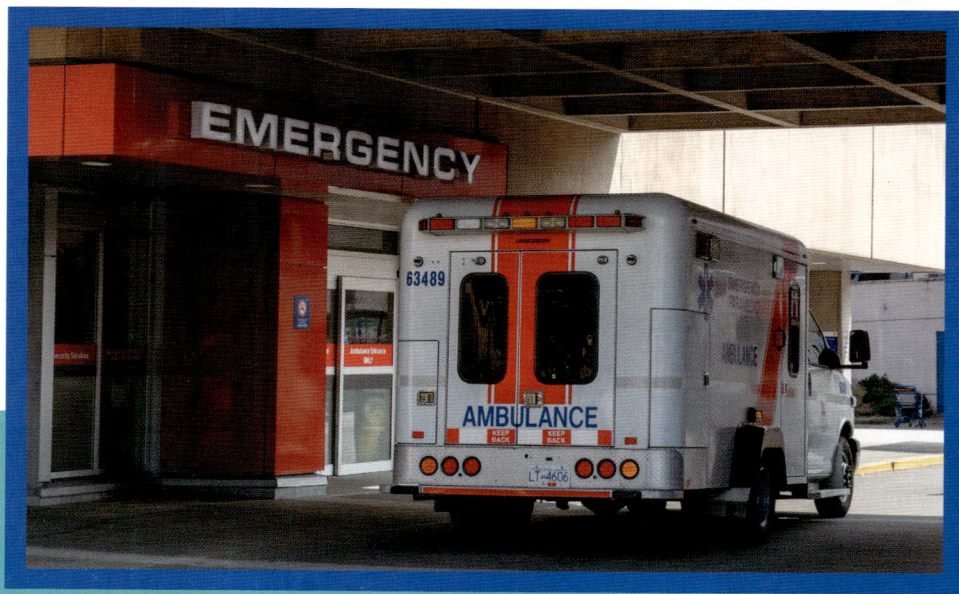

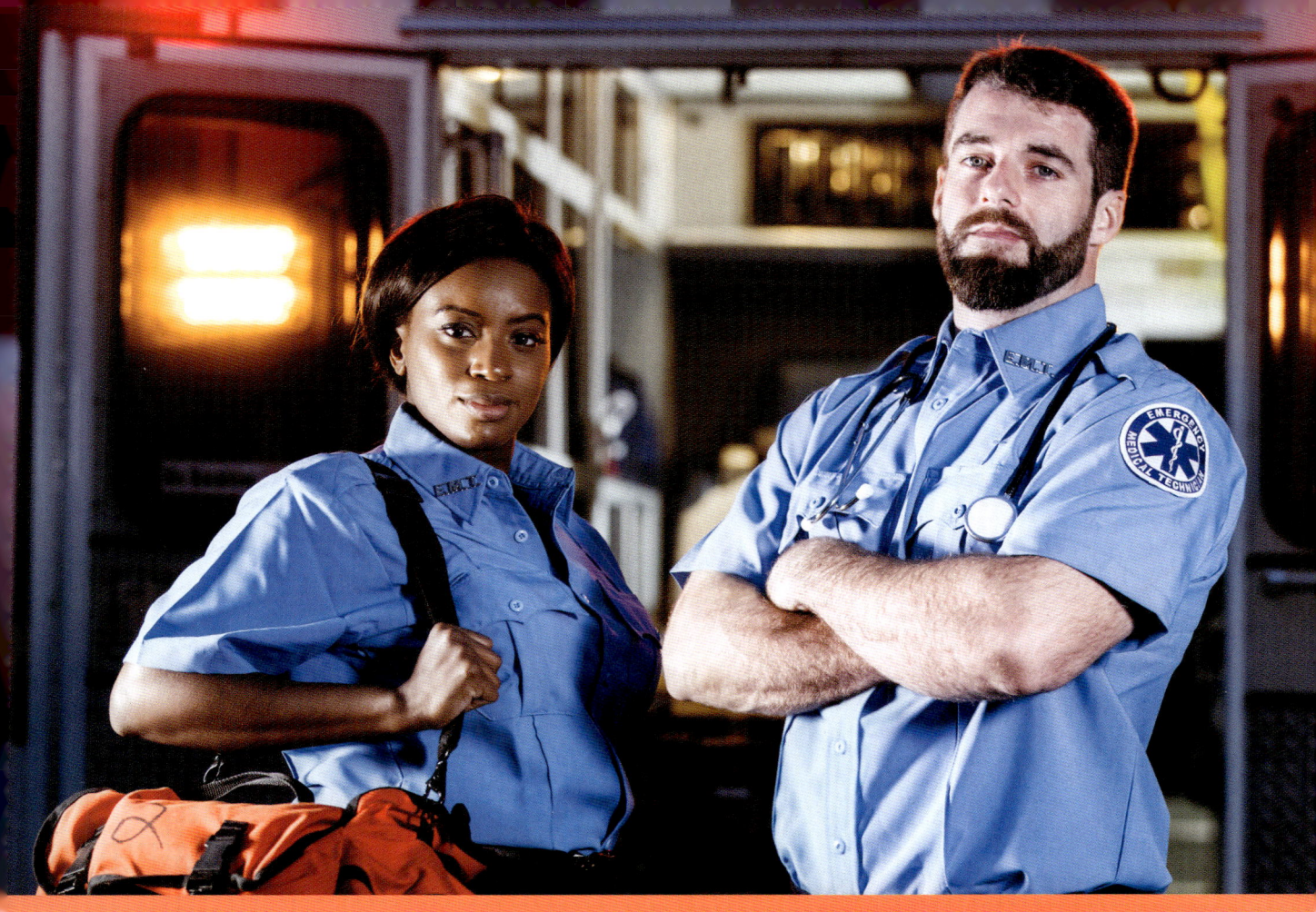

The sun sets. A new crew comes.
What will the night bring? No one knows.
But the ambulance will be ready!

AMBULANCE ARTWORK

You learned a lot about what ambulances do all day. Now you can design your own ambulance!

What You Need:

- sheet of paper
- colored pencils, pens, or crayons

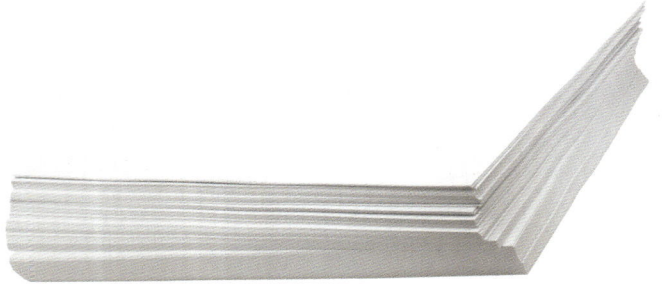

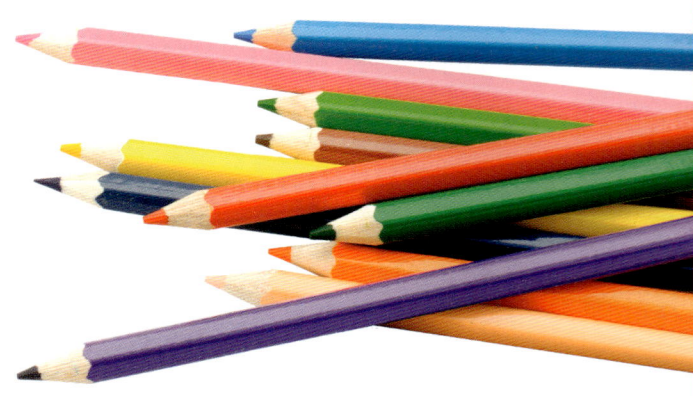

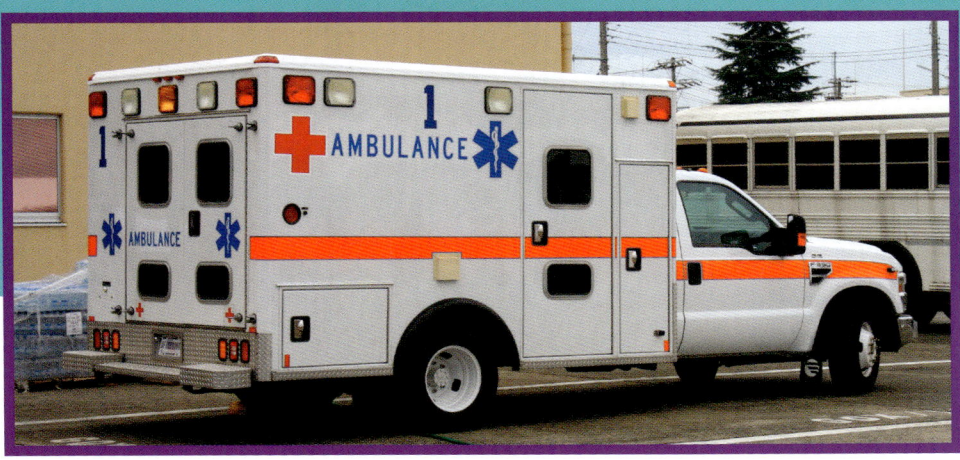

What You Do:

1. Draw an ambulance on a sheet of paper.

2. Add lights. You can draw medical symbols on the outside. For example, some ambulances have crosses on them. Others have a Star of Life. It is a six-pointed star. A rod with a snake around it is in the middle of the star.

3. Add ambulance workers into your drawing. You can add a patient too.

4. Share your drawing with your family and friends to show what you learned.

GLOSSARY

community (kuh-MYOO-nuh-tee)—a group of people who live in the same area

dispatcher (dis-PACH-uhr)—a person who answers emergency calls and sends rescue workers

emergency (i-MUHR-juhn-see)—a sudden and dangerous situation that must be handled quickly

emergency medical technician (i-MUHR-juhn-see MED-uh-kuhl tek-NI-shuhn)—a person trained to help people before and while being taken to a hospital

fuel (FEW-ul)—anything that can be burned to give off energy

paramedic (pa-ruh-MEH-dik)—a person trained to help people before and while being taken to a hospital; paramedics have more training than emergency medical technicians

patient (PAY-shunt)—a person who receives health care

stretcher (STRECH-ur)—a bed with straps and wheels that paramedics use to move patients

READ MORE

Bolte, Mari. *Important Jobs at Hospitals*. Mankato, MN: Capstone, 2023.

Brisson, Pat. *They're Heroes Too: A Celebration of Community*. Thomaston, ME: Tilbury House Publishers, 2022.

Sipperley, Keli. *Ambulances*. Mankato, MN: Capstone, 2022.

INTERNET SITES

Caroline County Department of Emergency Services: EMS for Kids
carolinemd.org/633/EMS-for-Kids

Kiddle: Ambulance Facts for Kids
kids.kiddle.co/Ambulance

Michigan Medicine: Explore the Inside of an Ambulance with This 360-Degree-Video
michiganmedicine.org/health-lab/explore-inside-ambulance-360-degree-video

INDEX

dispatchers, 12

emergency medical technicians (EMTs), 4

equipment checks, 10

fuel, 10

hospitals, 4, 6, 15, 17, 18

lights, 10, 13

paramedics, 4

patients, 7, 14, 15, 17, 18

stretchers, 8, 17, 18

ventilators, 8

ABOUT THE AUTHOR

Mae Respicio is a nonfiction writer and award-winning author of novels including *How to Win a Slime War*. Her dog, Riggs, loves to happily howl whenever he hears an emergency vehicle zoom by with its siren blaring!

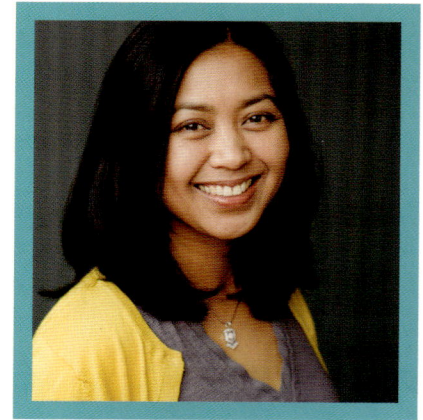